12 Days of Chair Yoga: For Seniors

Timothy J Smith CPT

12 Days of Chair Yoga

This simple guide will introduce you to the basic fundamental movements of Chair Yoga. Becoming familiar and comfortable with the basics will allow you to build a foundation that you can build upon as you progress in your self-improvement journey.

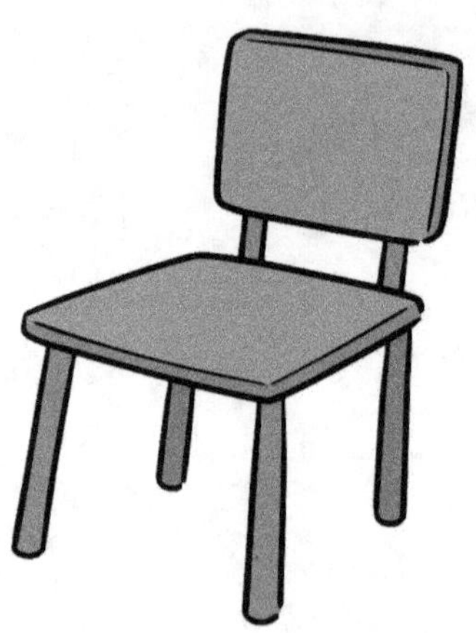

About the author

Timothy J Smith, CPT

With over 13 years of experience in the fitness realm, Timothy J Smith shares his knowledge with easily digestible daily bodyweight-only workout guides. Build a routine of consistent, new daily movements and workouts created by a Certified Personal Trainer from the National Academy Of Sports Medicine. Timothy's various titles in the Fitness Education/Personal Training category bring you multitudes of new programs to implement into your exercise routine. No matter your fitness level, you'll get your daily dose exercise in only 20 minutes or less- with no requirement for any gym equipment. Timothy J Smith is a Best-Selling personal fitness author as well as a Celebrity Personal Trainer based out of Beverly Hills, California. His experience in Private Personal-Training, Calisthenics, Senior training, and Recovery will be sure to help you level up your fitness.

Congrats on taking these steps to improve your life.

Timothy J Smith

Disclaimer:

Disclaimer: Before starting any new exercise routine, including chair yoga, it is advisable to consult with a qualified healthcare professional, such as a doctor or physical therapist. This precaution is particularly important if you have pre-existing health conditions, injuries, or concerns about your physical well-being. The information provided is not a substitute for professional medical advice, diagnosis, or treatment. Always seek the advice of your physician or another qualified health provider with any questions you may have regarding a medical condition. Discontinue any exercise that causes discomfort or exacerbates existing health issues, and seek prompt medical attention if needed.

Introduction to chair yoga

Chair yoga is a modified form of yoga that can be done while sitting on a chair or using a chair for support. It adapts traditional yoga poses and stretches to accommodate individuals with limited mobility or those who may find it challenging to practice yoga on the floor. The benefits of chair yoga include improved flexibility, strength, relaxation, and stress reduction. It's particularly beneficial for seniors, office workers, or anyone with physical limitations.

Chair yoga often incorporates gentle movements, deep breathing, and meditation techniques. It can enhance circulation, reduce joint strain, and promote better posture. The practice is adaptable, making it accessible for various fitness levels and ages. Additionally, chair yoga sessions are commonly used in workplaces to combat sedentary behavior and alleviate stress during the workday. It's important to consult with a healthcare professional before starting any new exercise routine, including chair yoga, especially if you have existing health concerns.

Recommendations

1) Use a sturdy chair on a non-slip surface such as carpet.

2) Focusing on proper form and technique is essential to avoiding injury.

3) Start slow and familiarize yourself with the basics before seeking to advance.

4) Lightly stretch before and after your yoga sessions to help with muscle recovery.

5) Aim to spend 15-20 minutes each day working on your movements.

6) If you feel tired, dizzy, or lightheaded, stop immediately and seek medical attention.

Let's Begin

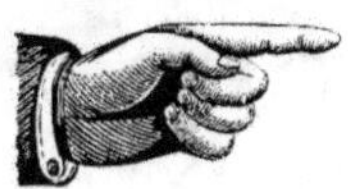 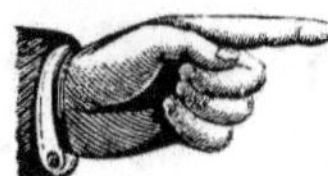 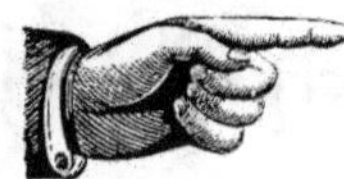

Pose #1:

Thigh Stretch

1) Stand behind your chair, lightly placing one hand on the backrest.

2) With your other hand, reach behind you and hold your foot in your hand with a light grip.

3) Stretch out your thigh muscles. Hold for 10-15 seconds before switching sides.

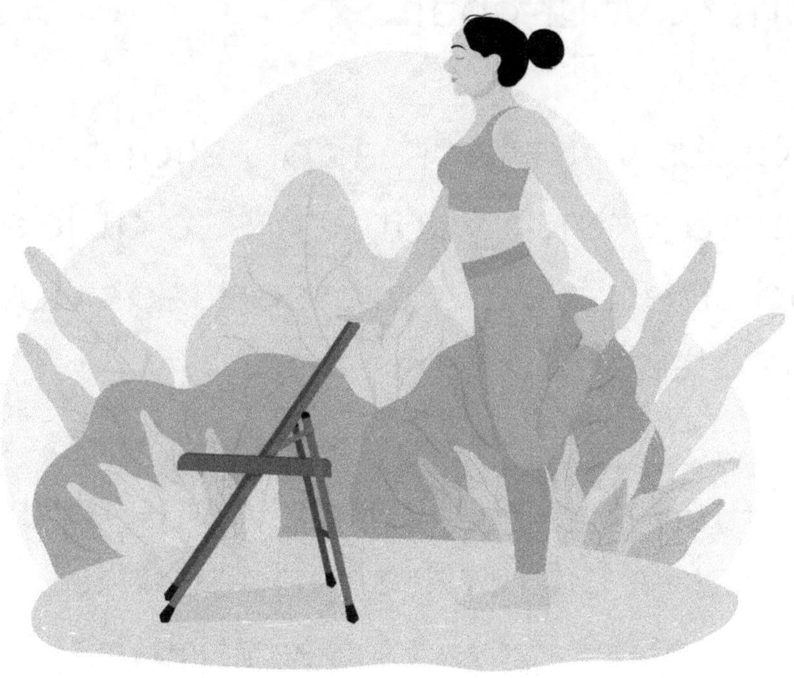

Thigh Stretch

Pose #2:

Lotus Pose

1) Sit flat on the ground beside or in front of your chair.

2) Cross your legs, apply slight pressure with your arms to guide and stretch your crossed legs down even-level with the floor.

3) Carefully and slowly work your stretch a bit further and further each time with a goal of becoming flexible enough in the groin and hip areas to assume this position almost effortlessly.

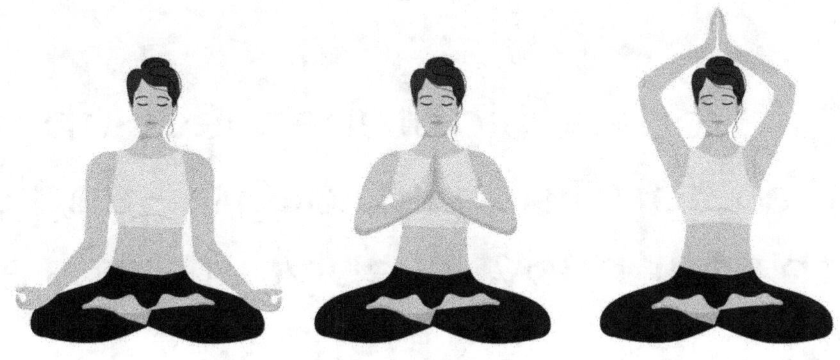

Lotus Pose

Pose #3:

Plow Pose

1) Lay flat on your back on the floor. Rest your arms at your sides and straighten your legs.

2) Lift your straightened legs up in the air, forming a 90 degree angle with your body. Keep your arms at your sides.

3) Keep your legs as straight as you can and perform 5-10 leg lifts.

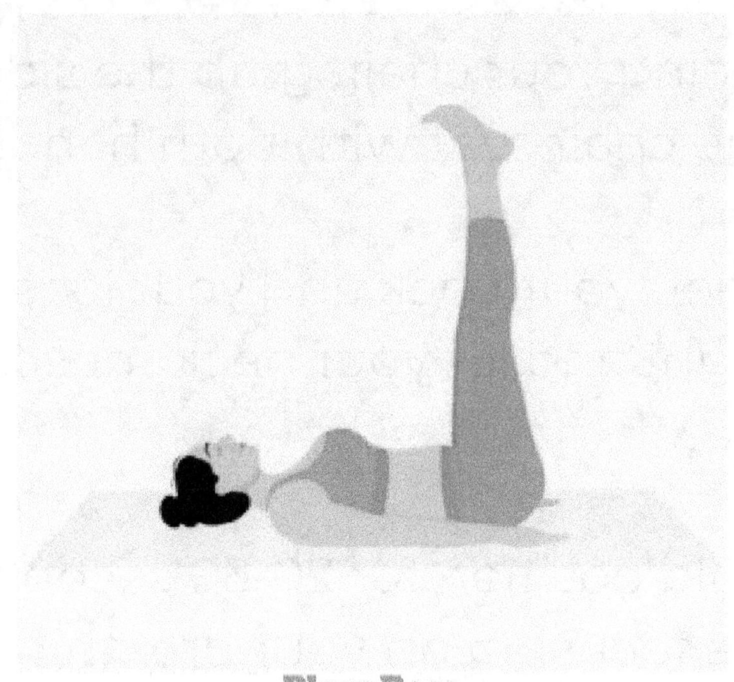

Plow Pose

Pose #4:

Chair Downward Dog

1) Facing your chair, grab the sides of the chair seat with both hands.

2) Keep your back and your legs straight and let your neck muscles relax.

3) Hold position for 20-30 seconds while focusing on your breathing.

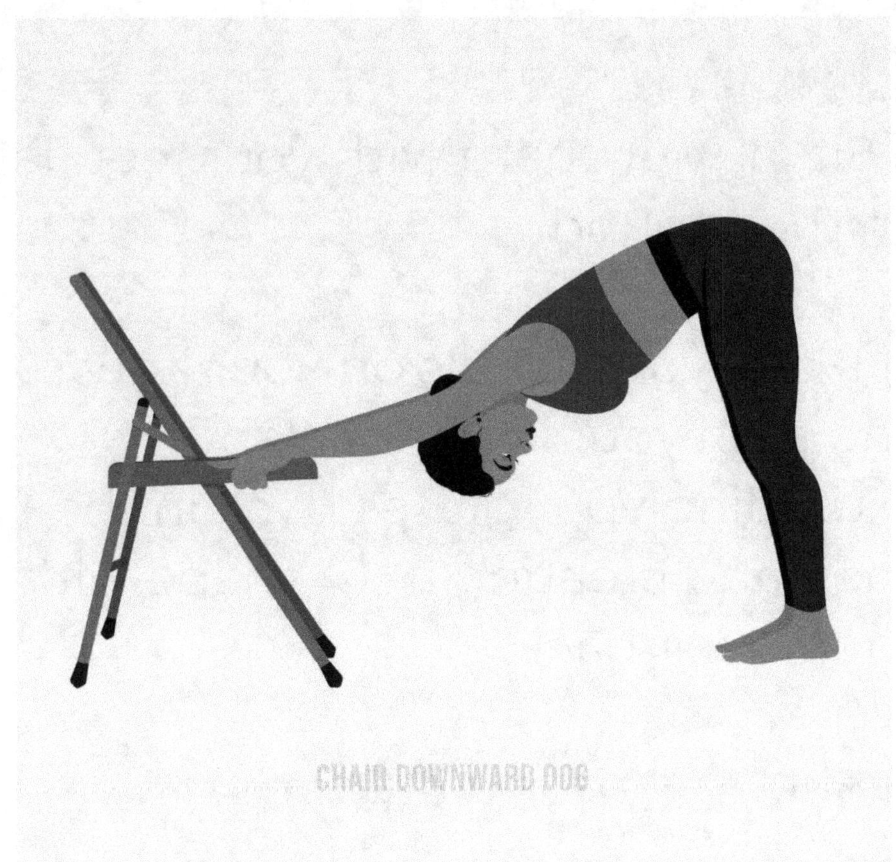
CHAIR DOWNWARD DOG

Pose #5:

Seated Cow

1) Sit in your share with your feet flat on the ground.

2) Place your hands on your knees and arch your lower back by extending your glutes back in the chair and creating a "C" shape with your lower back.

3) Slowly, perform 4-6 times.

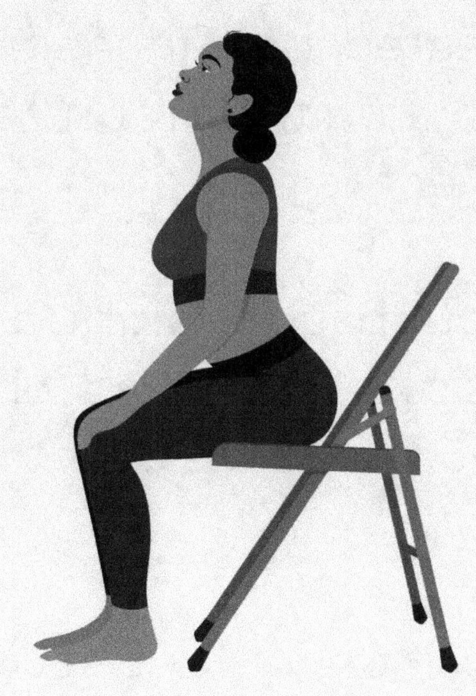

SEATED COW

Pose #6:

Seated Eagle

1) While seated in your chair, keep your feet flat on the ground and cross one leg over the other.

2) Keep your back straight, and raise your arms over your head while joining your forearms over top of one another.

3) Hold position for 10-15 seconds on each leg, and repeat the pose 3-5 times through.

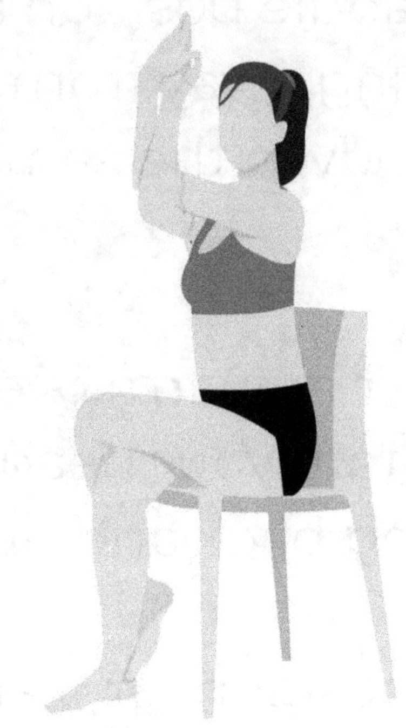

Seated Eagle

Pose #7:

Seated Extended Side Angle

1) Seated in your chair, move your legs to a straddle position and rotate one foot facing away from the chair. Face your body in the same direction as your foot.

2) Reach your rear arm over your body and rotate your head so that you're looking back and up in the air.

3) Hold the position for 10-15 seconds and then switch sides. Focus on stretching your muscles and controlling your breathing.

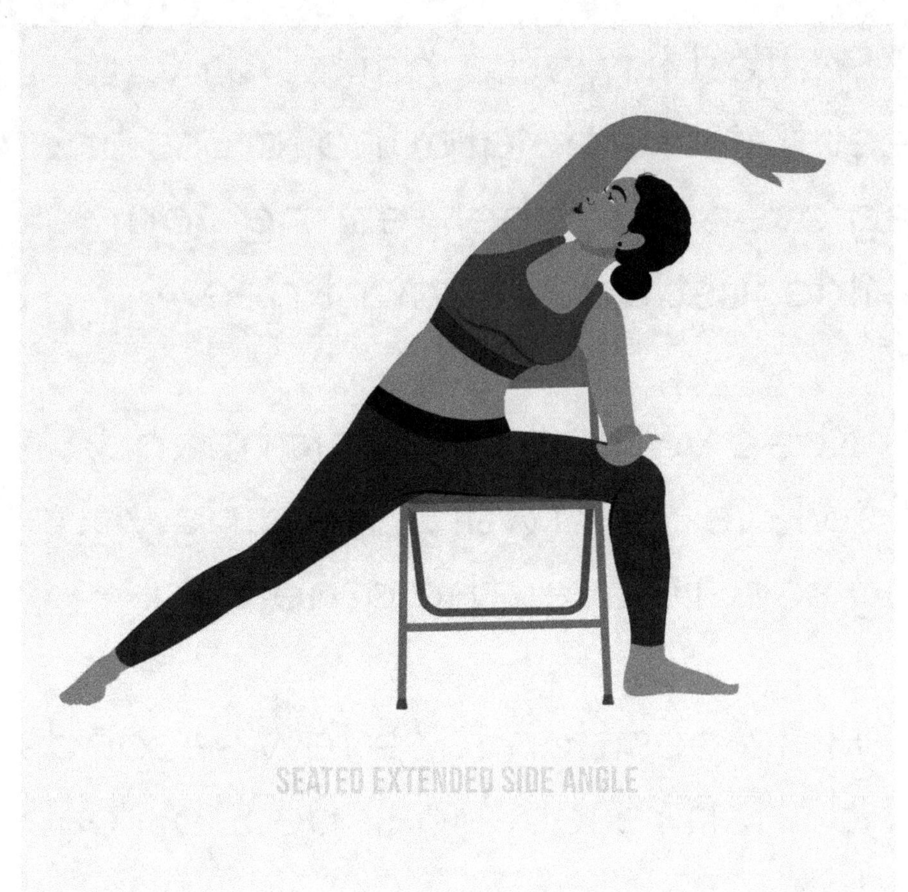

SEATED EXTENDED SIDE ANGLE

Pose #8:

Seated Pigeon

1) Seated in your chair with your feet flat on the ground, cross one leg over the other resting your ankle just above your knee.

2) Keep your back straight and slowly lean forward, holding your leg secure over the other leg.

3) Hold position for a few seconds and then reset and repeat on each side.

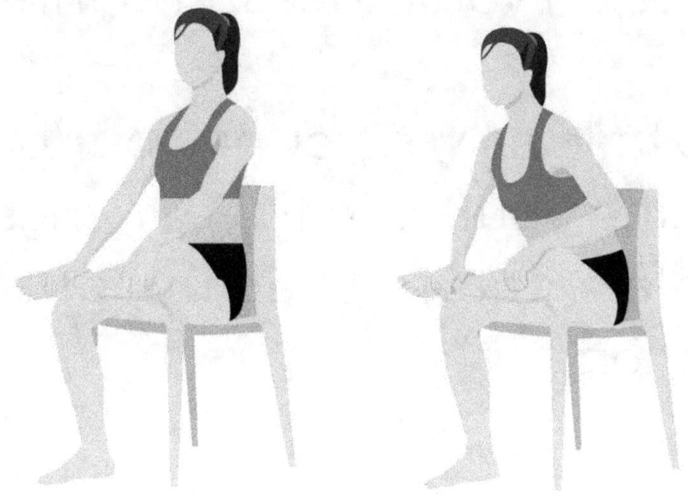

Seated Pigeon

Pose #9:

Seated Cat

1) Sit upright in a chair, place your hands on your knees, and inhale.

2) Exhale as you round your back, tucking your chin to your chest. Inhale to return to an upright position.

3) Repeat for a gentle seated cat stretch.

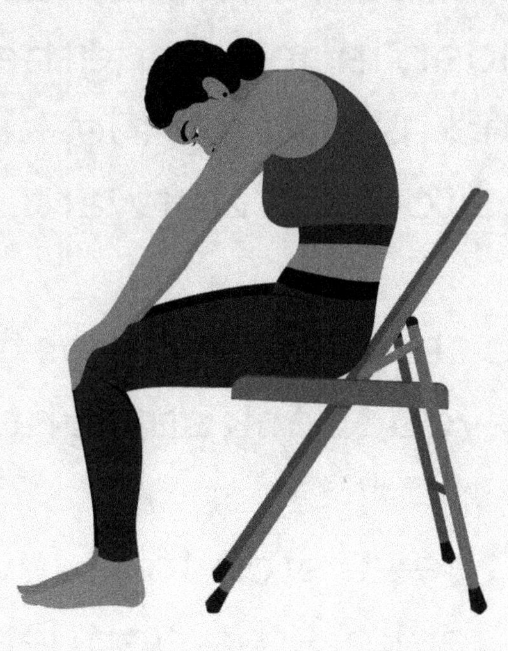

SEATED CAT

Pose #10:

Seated Forward Bend

1) Sit at the edge of a chair, feet flat on the floor. Inhale, lengthen your spine, and as you exhale, hinge at your hips to reach forward.

2) Hold onto your shins or feet, keeping your back straight.

3) Hold the stretch for a few breaths, feeling the gentle forward bend.

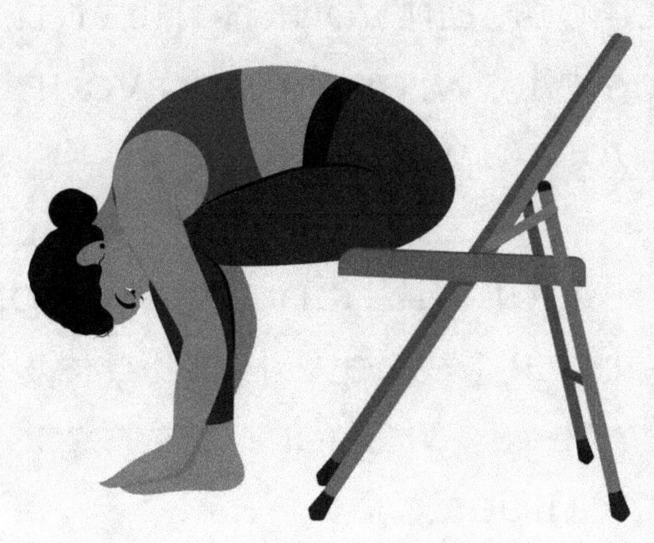

SEATED FORWARD BEND

Pose #11:

Shoulder Stretch

1) Sit tall in your chair with feet flat on the floor. Lift your right arm, bend it at the elbow, and bring your hand down your upper back.

2) With your left hand, gently press on your right elbow. Hold the stretch, feeling a gentle stretch in your shoulder.

3) Switch sides and repeat.

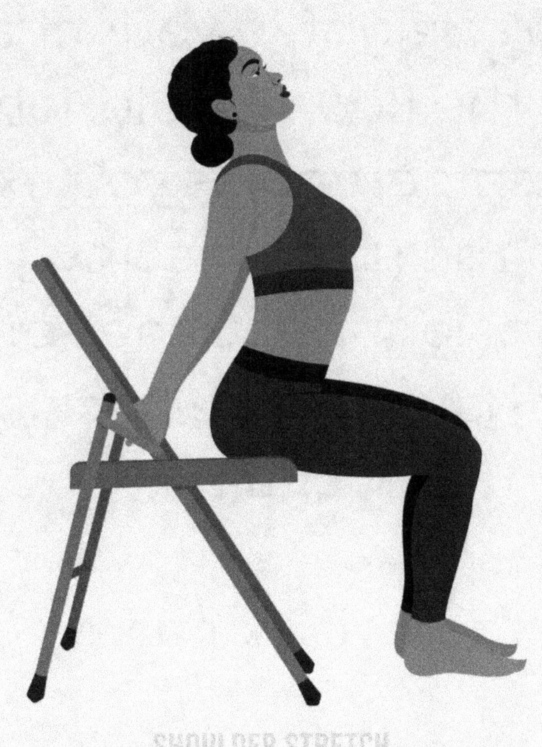

SHOULDER STRETCH

Pose #12:

Seated Easy Spinal Twist

1)Sit up straight in your chair, feet flat on the floor. Inhale, lengthen your spine, and as you exhale, twist to the right, placing your left hand on your right knee and your right hand on the back of the chair.

2) Hold the twist for a few breaths.

3) Return to the center and repeat on the other side.

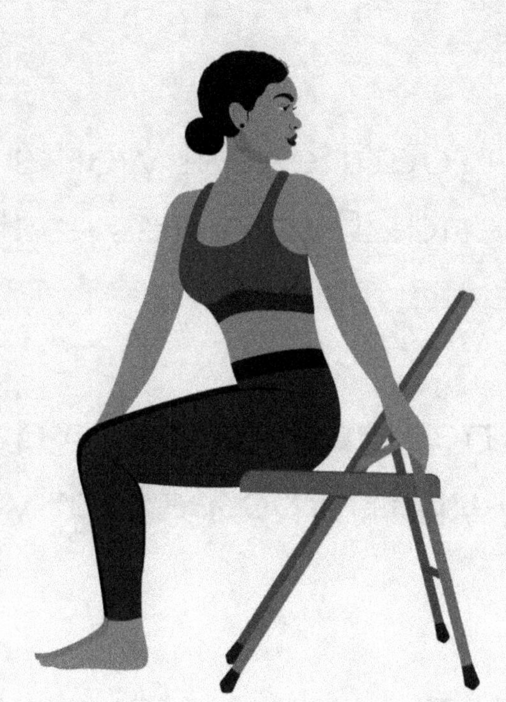

SEATED EASY SPINAL TWIST

Once you've gotten the basics down...

Try adding some variation and building a routine!

1) Create a routine that works for you. Aim to spend 20 minutes each day improving your form.

2) Build a new routine each day by switching up the poses that you practice.

3) Don't forget to maintain your flexibility. Just like anything else, constant practice yields progress. Stay consistent to achieve maximum results.

Know somebody that loves to put on muscle?

Check out:

"50 Days of Calisthenics Workouts"

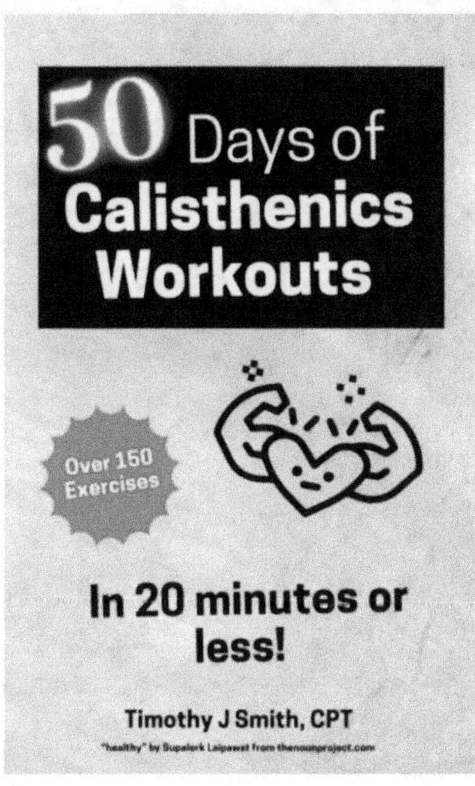

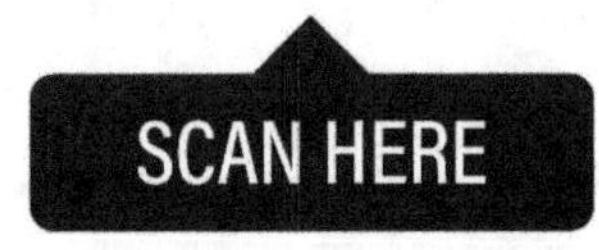

On Amazon!

Thanks for Reading!